IMMUNITY IGNITION

Therapies for Boosting the Immune System Naturally

Ignite Your Immune System With Natural Therapies And Lifestyle Practices To Enhance Overall Immunity

DR. BRIDGET PROMISE

Table of Contents

CHAPTER ONE

Introduction

Within the complex tapestry of existence, our immune system functions as an imperceptible guardian, ceaselessly exerting effort to fortify our body against external threats.

An intricate system comprising various cells, tissues, and organs functions as an intrinsic security apparatus, perpetually surveilling and safeguarding the body against detrimental pathogens. Gaining knowledge about the immune system and acknowledging the criticality of preserving its robustness are fundamental components in advocating for holistic wellness. This article provides an in-depth analysis of the immune system, emphasizing its significance and investigating natural methods to bolster and improve its operations.

A Comprehension Of The Immune System

An extraordinary feat of biological engineering, the immune system is comprised of an intricate network that works in concert to detect and eradicate extracellular substances, including pathogens, viruses, and toxins. The immune system, which consists of antibodies, white blood cells, and numerous other constituents, can be classified into two principal divisions: the innate immune system and the adaptive immune system.

The innate immune system functions as the primary barrier against pathogens, delivering prompt, non-specific reactions. It consists of chemical barriers, such as gastric acid, and physical barriers, such as the epidermis and mucous membranes.

In addition, numerous cells, including neutrophils and macrophages, serve as rapid responders for the body, consuming and neutralizing invaders.

Conversely, the adaptive immune system provides a response that is more precise and targeted. It acquires memory and "learns" from previous pathogen exposures, allowing for a more rapid and effective response to subsequent exposures. Lymphocytes, which are a subset of white blood cells, are essential for adaptive immunity. Antibodies are produced by B cells, while T cells attack infected cells directly.

The Critical Nature Of A Robust Immune System

Overall health maintenance and the prevention of infections and maladies require a robust immune system. It functions as a robust barrier, ceaselessly striving to detect and eliminate potential dangers, thus protecting the body against a multitude of diseases.

An optimally operating immune system is not solely essential for immediate defense, but also for sustained health using immunological memory formation.

A robust immune system is associated with an accelerated recuperation from diseases and mitigation of the intensity of symptoms in the event of infections.

Additionally, it serves as a critical component in the prevention of chronic diseases and specific forms of cancer through the detection and eradication of aberrant cells before their ability to proliferate.

In addition to safeguarding against pathogens, the immune system is involved in maintaining homeostasis and tissue repair. As a vital component of the immune response, inflammation aids in the restoration of damaged tissues and the resolution of infections.

Nevertheless, a chronic or hyperactive inflammatory response can result in a multitude of health complications, underscoring the importance of maintaining a delicate equilibrium to ensure optimal immune function.

Frequent Aspects Influencing Immunity

Numerous determinants can impact the robustness and

effectiveness of the immune system. How the body protects itself from external dangers is significantly influenced by environmental factors, personal health, and lifestyle decisions.

1. A nutrient-dense and well-balanced diet is essential for maintaining optimal immune health. Insufficiencies in vital vitamins and minerals, including selenium, vitamin C, vitamin D, and zinc, can impair the function of the immune system.

A diet abundant in fruits, vegetables, and other immune-boosting nutrients, on the contrary, can strengthen the immune system.

2. Chronic stress profoundly impairs the functionality of the immune system. The immune response can be suppressed by stress hormones like cortisol, rendering the body more vulnerable to infections. It is essential to exercise and incorporate stress-management techniques, such as meditation, to maintain a healthy equilibrium.

3. Sleep: Adequate sleep is fundamental to immune function and overall health. Critical bodily processes, including the release of

cytokines that regulate immune responses, occur during sleep. These processes may be compromised or disrupted due to insufficient or disturbed slumber, which may subsequently undermine the immune system.

4. Engaging in consistent physical activity enhances overall well-being, reduces inflammation, and promotes proper circulation, all of which are beneficial for maintaining a healthy immune system. Conversely, engaging in excessive or strenuous physical activity without sufficient rest can yield the reverse outcome—a

transient inhibition of immune functionality.

5. Hygiene and Environment: The immune system is strengthened through exposure to a diversity of microorganisms. Excessive reliance on antimicrobial products or an excessively sterilized environment may impede the development of a robust immune response. However, exposure to contaminants and pollutants can compromise the immune system's defenses.

CHAPTER TWO

Methods Utilizing Nature For Immune Support

Although genetics does contribute to the determination of immune function, habits, and behaviors have a substantial influence on its robustness. Adopting natural strategies for immune system support represents a proactive and holistic approach to improving one's overall health.

1. Nutritional Support: Eleventh-grade immune health is established upon the consumption of a balanced diet abundant in vitamins and minerals.

Antioxidant-rich foods, including almonds, verdant greens, and berries, can aid in the fight against oxidative stress and boost the immune system. Additionally, specific deficiencies may be remedied by supplementation when necessary, under the supervision of a healthcare professional.

2. Herbal Remedies: A multitude of herbs have exhibited immune-modulating characteristics and have been employed in traditional medicine for centuries. Herbs such as echinacea, elderberry, astragalus, and garlic are widely recognized for their purported

ability to bolster the immune system. By integrating these substances into one's regimen, be it via dietary supplements, beverages, or tinctures, supplementary immune support may be provided.

3. Probiotics: Immunity function is highly dependent on the gut microbiome, and a healthy balance of intestinal flora is essential for this. Probiotics, which are nutritional supplements and fermented foods such as yogurt, kefir, and sauerkraut, have the potential to positively impact the immune system and promote gastrointestinal health.

4. Consistent Physical Activity: Participating in moderate, routine exercise has been linked to improved immune function. Circulation is improved through physical activity, which permits immune cells to circulate freely throughout the body. Additionally, it aids in stress management and enhances overall immune resilience.

5. Ensuring that one has a substantial amount of high-quality sleep is a straightforward yet impactful method of bolstering the immune system. Stress management, the creation of a comfortable sleeping

environment, and the establishment of a regular sleep schedule are all factors that can positively impact restorative sleep and, as a result, the immune system.

In summary, gaining an appreciation for the intricate nature of the immune system, acknowledging its critical role in general health, and incorporating natural strategies to bolster its operation are fundamental measures in cultivating resilience and promoting overall wellness. Through the adoption of a holistic way of life, which includes proper nutrition, effective stress management, and the cultivation of healthy behaviors, individuals can enhance the functionality of their immune systems, thereby establishing a robust and resilient physical and mental fortitude.

Immunity And Dietary Health

The increasing significance of the intricate connection between immunity and nutrition stems from the desire of individuals to strengthen their defenses against a variety of diseases. The immune system is significantly aided by a well-balanced diet, which guarantees its optimal operation and receptivity to potential threats.

It is essential, in terms of nutrition and immune health, to consume an assortment of nutrient-dense foods. Fruits, vegetables, whole cereals, lean proteins, and nutritious lipids are included. A spectrum of vitamins, minerals, and antioxidants are provided by the synergistic effects of these dietary groups, all of which contribute to a healthy immune system.

Herbal Immune-Boosting Remedies

Herbal remedies, apart from conventional nutritional sources, have garnered attention due to their purported capacity to enhance the immune system. Herbs of diverse types have been utilized historically across cultures to promote immune function and general health for centuries.

An example of a widely recognized herb with immune-stimulating properties is Echinacea. According to scientific research, echinacea-derived compounds may bolster the functionality of immune cells, thereby assisting the body's immune response to infections.

Elderberry is another herb with potential immune-boosting properties. Elderberry, which is abundant in vitamins and antioxidants, has been linked to a diminished severity and duration of cold and flu symptoms. Anti-inflammatory properties are a contributing factor to its immune system-supporting efficacy.

Curcumin, an element found in turmeric, is frequently employed in traditional medicine. It possesses formidable antioxidant and anti-inflammatory properties. The anti-inflammatory and oxidative stress-reducing properties of turmeric may be enhanced through its supplementation or incorporation into the diet.

CHAPTER THREE

Vital Minerals And Vitamins For Immunity

Specific vitamins and minerals are essential for immune function support. Vitamin C is particularly noteworthy due to its antioxidant characteristics and its involvement in the synthesis and operation of white blood cells. Bell peppers, citrus fruits, and blueberries are all rich in vitamin C.

An additional essential nutrient that promotes optimal immune function is vitamin D. It is involved in the regulation of immune cell activity and the stimulation of antimicrobial peptide synthesis. Supplements, sun exposure, and dietary sources such as fortified products and fatty fish are common methods for ensuring adequate vitamin D intake.

Zinc, an indispensable mineral, facilitates the operation of immune cells, thereby bolstering the immune system. It is present in almonds, legumes, meat, dairy, and other nutrients. Immune function impairment has been linked to zinc deficiency, underscoring the criticality of maintaining optimal levels.

The Effects Of Physical Activity On The Immune System

Consistent engagement in physical activity is fundamental to maintaining a healthy lifestyle and offers numerous advantages, one of which is a beneficial influence on the immune system. Improved immune function has been associated with consistent, moderate exercise, which reduces the risk of chronic diseases and infections.

Physical activity facilitates the transportation of immune cells, thereby enhancing their capacity to identify and react to potential dangers. Furthermore, engagement in physical activity facilitates the secretion of endorphins, which have the potential to mitigate the detrimental effects of inflammation and stress on the immune system.

It is crucial to acknowledge that although moderate exercise can yield positive outcomes, engaging in excessive or intense training without sufficient recovery time may produce the opposite effect—a transient suppression of immune function. It is essential to maintain immune health by integrating rest and recovery into a fitness regimen and striking a balance.

The Importance Of Sound Sleep For Immune Health

The importance of adequate sleep in promoting immune function cannot be emphasized enough. Sleep is an essential period for bodily restoration and regeneration; therefore, sleep pattern disturbances can weaken the immune system.

The body produces cytokines, which are proteins that are essential for immune response, inflammation, and healing, while at rest. A compromised immune response and a decrease in cytokine production may result from sleep deprivation.

A prolonged recuperation period following illness and an increased susceptibility to infections have been linked to chronic sleep deprivation. It is critical to prioritize good sleep hygiene, establish consistent sleep schedules, and create a conducive sleep environment to promote immune function and overall health.

Through the integration of a varied and nourishing dietary regimen, investigation into the potential advantages of herbal remedies, acquisition of sufficient quantities of immune-supporting vitamins and minerals, participation in consistent and well-balanced physical activity, and prioritization of high-quality sleep, individuals can enhance the functionality of their immune systems, thereby fostering holistic health and fortitude against adversity.

CHAPTER FOUR

Techniques For Stress Management To Preserve An Immune System

In addition to being advantageous for mental health, stress management is crucial for maintaining a healthy immune system.

The gradual suppression of the immune response can occur as a result of stress hormones, including cortisol, that are secreted in response to chronic stress. To mitigate this, it is critical to integrate stress management techniques into one's daily routine.

1. Consistently participating in mindfulness and meditation exercises has been demonstrated to alleviate tension and foster a state of tranquility. By training the mind to concentrate on the present moment, these techniques enable people to escape the cycle of tension and anxiety. The efficiency of the immune system can increase as stress levels decrease.

2. Engaging in regular physical activity not only serves as a tension reliever but also

contributes to the maintenance of optimal health. Activation stimulates the secretion of endorphins, which are endogenous mood enhancers and aids in the regulation of stress hormones. A regime consisting of a variety of physical activities—including aerobic exercise, strength training, and flexibility exercises—contributes to an enhanced immune system.

3. Sufficient Sleep: Sleep of high quality is vital for one's overall health, which includes immune function. The immune system can be compromised by chronic sleep deprivation, rendering the body

more vulnerable to infections. By adhering to a regular sleep schedule and guaranteeing a minimum of seven to nine hours of uninterrupted sleep per night, one can enhance their immune resilience.

The Function Of Hydration In Aiding Immunity

Although frequently disregarded, adequate hydration is a critical component in bolstering the immune system. Water is an essential nutrient for the proper operation of numerous physiological processes, including those that support immune health.

1. Immune Function and Hydration: Maintaining adequate hydration is critical for the circulation and secretion of lymph, the fluid that transports immune cells throughout the body. Impairment of the lymphatic system due to dehydration may impede the immune response. Consistently consuming sufficient water is essential for preserving the equilibrium required for optimal immune functionality.

2. Herbal Teas and Infusions: Herbal teas and infusions, when combined with ordinary water, have the potential to offer supplementary immune-boosting

advantages. Herbal infusions containing substances such as chamomile, echinacea, and ginger support the immune system. These beverages serve the dual purpose of promoting hydration and enhancing overall well-being through their flavorful qualities.

The Interplay Between the Gut and Immune System: Cultivating a Stable Microbiome

A complex community of microorganisms residing in the digestive tract, the gut microbiome is essential for immune function regulation. An equitable and varied microbiome is a factor in the development of a robust immune system.

1. The incorporation of probiotics into one's dietary regimen, be it via dietary supplements or fermented foods such as sauerkraut, yogurt, and kefir, facilitates the proliferation of advantageous bacteria within the gastrointestinal tract. By regulating the environment and inhibiting the proliferation of pathogenic microorganisms, these bacteria bolster the immune system.

2. Adherence to a high-fiber diet promotes gastrointestinal health

through the provision of sustenance for beneficial flora. Legumes, fruits, vegetables, and whole grains are all outstanding sources of fiber. Optimal gastrointestinal health is a factor in a heightened immune response.

Holistic Methods To Promote Immune Health

Holistic approaches to immune wellness transcend particular symptoms by attending to the body's and mind's equilibrium as a whole.

1. Herbal Supplements: It can be advantageous to include herbal supplements, such as astragalus,

echinacea, and elderberry, which are recognized for their potential to enhance the immune system. It is crucial, nevertheless, to seek the advice of a healthcare professional before incorporating supplements into your daily regimen.

2. Acupuncture and Traditional Medicine: Originating in traditional medicine, acupuncture and similar techniques seek to restore energy balance to the body. It is believed that these holistic approaches promote well-being in its entirety, including immune function.

CHAPTER FIVE

Investigating Mind-Body Therapies To Boost The Immune System

The interrelation between the psyche and body exerts a significant impact on immune function and general well-being. The objective of mind-body therapies is to utilize this connection to promote health.

1. Yoga and Tai Chi are mind-body disciplines that integrate breathing regulation, meditation, and physical postures. Engaging in these activities has been linked to

a decrease in stress levels and an improvement in immune function.

2. Breathwork and Deep Relaxation Techniques: The body's relaxation response can be triggered by performing deliberate breathwork, such as deep diaphragmatic breathing or guided relaxation exercises. These techniques aid in the mitigation of stress and bolster the resilience of the immune system.

Finally, it can be stated that a robust immune system can be substantially enhanced by emphasizing stress management, adequate hydration, a balanced intestinal microbiome, and holistic practices. By integrating these strategies into their everyday routines, people can enhance their bodies' ability to protect themselves from external hazards, resulting in an overall state of wellness. Bear in mind that developing a robust immune system requires attending to both the mental and physical dimensions of health.

Factors In The Environment And Immune Health

The correlation between environmental factors and immune health is an essential component in the preservation of holistic wellness. The immune system, which is comprised of an intricate network of proteins and cells, is critical for protecting the body from pathogens, bacteria, and viruses. Gaining knowledge regarding the impact of environmental factors on immune health enables individuals to make well-informed decisions that bolster the body's innate defense mechanisms.

An assortment of environmental factors, including the oxygen we breathe, the food we consume, and our lifestyle decisions, can affect immune function. By incorporating natural immune-boosting recipes, strategic meal plans, and targeted supplements into one's diet, it is possible to bolster the body's resistance to infections and diseases.

Menus And Natural Immune-Boosting Recipes

Adhering to a nutritious diet is essential for sustaining a strong immune system. Meal plans and recipes that include immune-boosting ingredients may contain the nutrients required to support immune function. Important components include:

1. Vibrant fruits and vegetables, which are abundant in

antioxidants, vitamins, and minerals, are an essential component of a balanced immune-boosting diet. Bell peppers, spinach, asparagus, berries, and citrus fruits are all excellent options.

2. Protein is a fundamental component that ensures the effective operation of immune cells. Include lean protein sources in your diet, such as poultry, fish, legumes, and tofu.

3. When deciding what to eat, choose whole grains like quinoa, brown rice, and oats. These foods offer a consistent supply of vital

nutrients and vitality, thereby promoting overall well-being.

4. Incorporate nutritious lipids into your diet, such as avocados, almonds, and olive oil. Insulin regulation and fat-soluble vitamin absorption are both facilitated by these lipids.

5. Foods abundant in probiotics, such as yogurt, kefir, and sauerkraut, comprise advantageous microorganisms that promote gastrointestinal well-being. Strong immune function is intricately connected to gastrointestinal health.

By organizing meals according to these principles, one can guarantee a varied and nourishing consumption that furnishes the body with the necessary resources to operate at its highest level.

Supplements To Help The Immune System

Although maintaining a balanced diet is essential, bolstering immune health with supplements can be particularly beneficial in cases where particular nutrients are in short supply. Important supplements consist of:

1. Vitamin C is well-known for its ability to enhance the immune

system by promoting the development and operation of white blood cells. It also protects cells from injury by functioning as an antioxidant.

2. Vitamin D is a critical nutrient for immune function as it supports the body's defense against infections and helps regulate the immune response. While sunlight exposure is a natural source of vitamin D, supplementation may be required in areas with limited sunlight, in particular.

3. Zinc is an essential mineral for immune cell development and function. Supplemental zinc can

be advantageous, particularly for those who are deficient in this element.

4. Elderberry extract, which is widely utilized for its antiviral properties, may aid in reducing the severity and duration of colds and influenza.

5. Probiotics, when taken in the form of supplements, have the potential to support a healthy intestinal microbiome and exert a beneficial impact on immune function.

CHAPTER SIX

Modifications To One's Lifestyle That Promote Immune Resilience Over Time

In addition to dietary patterns and dietary supplements, lifestyle decisions have a substantial influence on immune resilience. Implementing the following simple adjustments into one's daily routine may have a lasting positive impact on immune health:

1. Sufficient sleep is an essential component for maintaining optimal immune system function. Aim for seven to nine hours of

sleep per night to facilitate repair and regeneration of the body.

2. Consistent and moderate physical activity enhances immune function through the promotion of healthy circulation and the mitigation of inflammation. Participate in enjoyable activities, such as yoga, cycling, or walking.

3. Chronic stress has the potential to exert detrimental effects on the immune system. To mitigate tension, integrate into your daily regimen stress-relieving activities such as mindfulness, deep breathing exercises, or meditation.

4. Maintaining adequate hydration is critical for one's overall health. Water facilitates nutrient transport, contaminant elimination, and the maintenance of optimal bodily functions.

5. It is advisable to abstain from smoking and excessive alcohol consumption, as both can have detrimental effects on immune function. Reducing one's alcohol intake and quitting smoking are both beneficial for one's overall health and immune system resilience.

6. Adherence to routine hygiene practices, such as consistent

handwashing, can effectively impede the transmission of infections. Maintaining good hygiene is critical for preserving immune health.

In Conclusion, Enhancing The Body's Inherent Defense Mechanisms

In summary, by comprehending and mitigating the impact of environmental factors on immune health, individuals are empowered to assert authority over their condition. Supplements that target the immune system, natural recipes that bolster the immune system, and strategic meal plans are all essential components in supplying the body with the critical capabilities to combat pathogens.

Including practical modifications to one's lifestyle additionally fortifies long-term immune resilience. Sufficient sleep, consistent physical activity, effective stress management, adequate hydration, and the adoption of healthy behaviors are all components of a holistic well-being regimen that bolsters the immune system's ongoing defense mechanisms.

Through the use of well-informed decisions regarding diet,

supplements, and lifestyle, individuals can actively enhance the potency and effectiveness of their immune system. Adopting a proactive stance towards immune health signifies a commitment to sustained welfare, as it fosters a resilient defense against infections and contributes to an overall healthier and more resilient existence.